Erectile Dysfunction: Combat Impotence with Effective Natural Solutions

By: Nick Stanton

Published by:

Nick Stanton and Random Technologies

4409 HOFFNER AVENUE, SUITE 347

Belle Isle, FL 32812

www.MensGrowth.com

Disclaimer

Table of Contents

Introduction

Erectile dysfunction (or impotence) is one of the more embarrassing ailments in which men will face in their lives, and is a major source of anxiety amongst sufferers.

Erectile dysfunction is defined as an individual's inability to develop or maintain a penile erection for satisfactory sexual intercourse.

The condition is common in America, with somewhere between 15-30 million men affected. However, with the appropriate treatment (which might psychotherapy, drug therapy, vacuum devices, and surgery) it is treatable.

This subject is often ignored due to the extreme sensitivity and the negative psychological connotations associated with erectile and sexual issues.

About this Report

The report that follows is a collection of important information about the disease and the best ways in which to fight it. Please take the time to read through the whole document. This gives you the best opportunity to reduce your pain and to hasten your return to full health. The report contains the following sections:

Chapter 1: Overview of Erectile Dysfunction/Impotence. Discusses what Erectile Dysfunction is, what causes it, who is at risk, how it is diagnosed, what the signs and symptoms are and the typical complications associated with erectile dysfunction.

Chapter 2: Conventional Erectile Dysfunction Remedies. Discusses traditional medical remedies.

Chapter 3: Alternative Treatment & Natural Remedies. Discusses alternative remedies and treatments that you can easily provide for yourself in your own home.

Chapter 4: Summary. Discusses your role in your overall health and contemplates what opportunities a healthy lifestyle will afford you.

In addition, reference materials for information, links and resources are included.

Please note: The words impotence and dysfunction are synonymous, and therefore interchangeable in the context of this report.

Erectile Dysfunction and Impotence:

Overview

Our first chapter, we'll look at the origins of erectile dysfunction, essentially what is it and what causes it. The first step in treating any condition is to understand the affects it can have on the body and the treatment options available. As we're often told visualization and a willingness to fight a condition is extremely helpful in the long term, and this report will empower you to start a healthier you.

What is it?

Quite simply, sexual dysfunction in men relates to difficulties in performing sexual intercourse. The most common form of sexual dysfunction is erectile dysfunction, caused by physical or psychological issues. The difficulty in any treatment plans is that the cause can occur through a combination of those issues and the physical causes can often create or worsen physiological fears. Physiological factors can include stress, fear, anxiety and performance pressures. The last of which is an incredibly troublesome issue to overcome and further prevents some men from enjoying sexual intercourse.

Normal Sexual Function

Despite what movies and popular culture tell us, sexual intercourse is not simple. Normal intercourse intricate movements in the body and complex functions of the brain as thoughts, memories and emotions are recycled and active.

Because the nervous, circulatory and endocrine (hormonal) systems all interact with the mind to produce a sexual response, the result is much more interrelated than we imagine. Interestingly, and a point we'll touch on later in this report, the sexual response in men is largely driven by the nervous system.

Normal sexual function emanates from desire (also called sex drive or libido), which is the want to engage in sexual activity. Desire can be triggered by words, sights, smells and touch, and leads to the first stage of the sexual response cycle, excitement. Excitement is sexual arousal, and during such phase, blood flow to the penis increases (as does muscle tension throughout the body), leading to an erection.

Sexual intercourse can result in orgasm, defined as the peak or climax of sexual excitement. At orgasm, the muscle tension already at a heightened state increases further, which in men, means an increased contraction rate in the pelvic muscles resulting in ejaculation (usually involving a release of semen, but not always). Although the two usually occur at the same time, they are indeed separate events and ejaculation can occur without orgasm and vice versa (although this may depend on the individual's stage of life (e.g. pre pubescent) or the use of drugs).

After orgasm, men immediately return to a non-aroused state and struggle to regain an erection for some time. Again, this may depend on the age of the individual, as the actual time may be shorter for younger men (e.g. the time between erections generally increases as men age).

What Causes Impotence?

Psychological Causes of Sexual Dysfunction:
- Anger towards a partner;
- Anxiety;
- Depression;
- Discord or boredom with a partner
- Fear of pregnancy, dependence on another person, or losing control;

- Feeling of detachment from sexual activities or one's partner;
- Guilt;
- Inhibitions or ignorance about sexual behavior;
- Performance anxiety (worrying about performance during intercourse); and
- Previous traumatic sexual experiences (for example, rape, incest, sexual abuse, or previous sexual dysfunction).

How is Erectile Dysfunction Different to Intercourse?

In the context of normal sexual intercourse described above, erectile dysfunction is the inability to get and maintain an erection. Although, all men will at times struggle to achieve an erection, dysfunction is only a concern for those that struggle on an ongoing and consistent basis.

The issue can be both severe and mild, with the determining factors as to which level an individual has dependent on how difficult it is to achieve an erection, how difficult it is to maintain an erection, and whether the erection is suitable for penetration. An individual with severe dysfunction will rarely be able to gain an erection.

Erectile dysfunction increases with age. Almost three quarters of those over 80 suffer from it and approximately half of those over 65.

The Medical Reasons

The basis of an erection is the adequate inflow of blood flow and at the same time a slowing of the blood outflow.

Therefore, disorders that narrow arteries and decrease blood flow (such as atherosclerosis, diabetes or a blood clot) are physical reasons that can cause erectile dysfunction. In the same sense, abnormalities with the veins of the penis can drain blood away from the penis preventing erections from being maintained.

Another cause of dysfunction is neurological damage. Understandably, damage to the nerves leading to or from the penis will also prevent the achievement of an erection. The damage could be caused by surgery (most commonly prostate surgery), spinal disease, diabetes, multiple sclerosis, peripheral nerve disorders, a stroke, or the excessive use of alcohol and drugs.

The physical causes of the condition can also include hormonal disturbances (such as abnormally low levels of testosterone). This particular cause is heavily linked with factors affecting individual's energy levels, meaning factors such as illness; stress; and fatigue can play a part in the ability to gain an erection.

Additionally, drugs can interfere with sexual intercourse and erections. Research has found that antihypertensives, antidepressants, some sedatives, cimetidine, digoxin, lithium and antipsychotics can have a negative reaction with the body and work against the body's attempts to achieve an erection.

Aside from the physical causes of the damaging condition, psychological issues too (such as depression, performance anxiety, guilt, fear of intimacy and ambivalence about sexual orientation) can prevent an individual's ability to maintain an erection. Unlike physical factors, psychological causes are more common in younger men. This is evident in performance anxiety associated with a first sexual experience, a change of sexual partner, problems in a relationship or career stress.

Symptoms of Erectile Dysfunction and Impotence

The symptoms of an inability to raise an erection or no longer having erections during sleep or upon awakening are relatively obviously given the physical response of the body, however there are other symptoms of the condition.

The first additional symptom is the loss of sex drive (libido), which can mean that an erection (if achieved) may not be sufficiently hard, may not be sufficiently elevated or may subside before penetration can occur. This may result in strong erections at some times but trouble attaining or maintain erections other times.

With low testosterone this issue can be heightened and is likely to result in a drop in sex drive. Additionally, low testosterone levels can eventuate in the gradual development of many symptoms including enlargement of breast tissue (gynecomastia), raised pitch of the voice, shrinking of testes (testicles) and loss of muscle mass.

How is it Diagnosed?

In order to diagnose erectile dysfunction a doctor must perform a proper medical examination of the patient's genitals but also look to some of the causes and symptoms above to appreciate the full reasons behind the impotence. Because other issues could include issues with nerves and blood vessels a full assessment of the patients overall heath and arteries is required.

To assist in the diagnosis a blood sample is required to measure the levels of testosterone in the patient's blood. These samples also help to identify whether the patient is at risk of diabetes, which can cause problems with erectile dysfunction, whether permanent or temporary.

Lastly, an ultrasound may be needed if the doctor suspects' complications caused in the arteries or veins. An ultrasound will help reveal any such blockages within the penis.

Available Treatments for Erectile Dysfunction and Impotence

Not all affected men will bother to seek treatment for their dysfunction issues. For them the love of their partner and the ability to create physical connections in other ways may suffice and supersede the need for treatment.

However, the improvements made in the treatment of erectile dysfunction have seen an increase in the number of men seeking treatment. Some of the techniques used to treat the impotency, with detail to follow, include suppositories, injectable medication, implants and vacuum devices.

CONVENTIONAL DRUG TREATMENTS

Testosterone Replacement Therapy

At the age of 30 the levels of testosterone in men starts to reduce by 1-2% per year. This reduction in testosterone is akin to menopause in women but is by no means the same despite often being called male menopause. That occurs more rapidly and is nearly universal.

Low testosterone levels can lead to decreased libido, decreased muscle mass, increased abdominal fat, thin bones that easily fracture, decreased energy level, slow mathematical and spatial thinking and a low red blood cell count.

Thus a large number of men with low testosterone levels attempt to slow or reverse the reaction by taking testosterone. Unfortunately this is only effective in men with abnormally low levels of testosterone.

Complications of Testosterone Replacement Therapy

Although, testosterone replacement therapy can counteract the problems associated with the problems of low levels of testosterone, it can come with some worrying side effects. The worst side effect is unquestionably the risk of prostate disease. Most men develop a form of prostate cancer so small and dormant that it is not an issue, but the testosterone and unnatural levels can make the cancer grow, potentially to a lethal level. Testosterone also worsens benign prostatic hyperplasia, a non-cancerous enlargement of the prostate.

Therefore, this type of replacement therapy is only recommended for patients without signs of the disease, and those who are undertaking the treatment need to be checked regularly. The tests can often help in the detection and early prevention of the cancers.

Testosterone therapy is not a measure to increase blood flow to the penis. Rather, it works by correcting the hormonal balance to re-sustain abnormally low testosterone levels. Replacement can be achieved in many forms including pills, patches, topical creams, and injections, with most of them sharing similar side effects from liver dysfunction and increased red blood cell counts, through to an increased risk of stroke and enlargement of the prostate.

Other Drug Treatments

A range of drugs are available to treat erectile dysfunction, most of which increase blood flow the penis. More often than not the drugs are taken orally, but in rare cases are injected directly into the penis.

The most common drug on the market is Sildenafil. Sildenafil, an oral drug, increases the frequency and rigidity of erections within 30 to 60 minutes, if (and only if) the man is aroused. Erections tend to last about 10 to 30 minutes, but the drug can come with some side effects. On the minor scale these can include headaches, flushes, runny nose, upset stomach, and vision problems, and on the more serious side the drug can cause dangerously low blood pressure when taken with certain other drugs (such as nitroglycerin or amyl nitrite). Men should never take Sildenafil with other drugs such as nitroglycerin and if they have any concerns about the ingredients of other medicine should seek the advice of a professional.

Other oral drugs that have been used in the treatment of erectile dysfunction are Phentolamine, Yohimbine, and testosterone. Phentolamine is less effective than Sildenafil while Yohimbine is mainly used for psychological effects. Yohimbine can cause anxiety, shaking, rapid heart rate, and increased blood pressure) and is accordingly less effective than both of the above options.

All of the drugs mentioned thus far are taken orally, which can mean those who are unable to take drugs in their mouth must use alternative methods such as injection for treatments.

A second drug that is also not taken orally is the drug Alprostadil. It is taken in the form of a pellet (suppository) that is inserted into the urethra of the penis. When used independently, Alprostadil can result in erections, but it is much more effective when used in conjunction with another treatment, such as a binding device. Side effects such as light-headedness, a burning sensation of the penis or painful erections can result from the use of Alprostadil.

Complications of Drug Treatments

Priapism

In basic terms, priapism is a prolonged and painful erection that can last from several hours up to a few days. Contrary to popular belief, this condition is not associated with sexual desire.

In the normal erection process blood flows into the penis and, usually following an orgasm, drains out of the penis without discomfort. When priapism occurs the blood is unable to drain as it would normally. The penis is therefore stagnate and remains erect. Priapism is usually always caused by the drug the individual takes to gain an erection, but in rare instances can be caused by medical conditions such as leukemia.

Symptoms of Priapism

In contrast to a normal erection, priapism lasts longer (usually hours) is not accompanied by sexual arousal and is exceptionally painful. The penis may also softer than a normal, but the underlying symptom will indefinitely be the pain.

The first stage of treatment is to stop the use of any drug that could be causing the priapism. Next an injection directly into the penis with a drug that can reduce the effect of the erection is recommended (for example, epinephrine, phenylephrine, terbutaline, or ephedrine), or a spinal anesthetic if the spinal cord seems to be the root cause. If a blood clot is the potential cause, surgery is necessary to restore normal circulation in the penis.

If these treatments do not return the penis to a flaccid state, it may be necessary to drain the blood from the penis with a needle and syringe. Doing so can also remove blood clots or blockages in the vessels.

A combination of the treatments above could be used but individual results may vary. It is also important to note that prolonged priapism usually impairs erectile function on a permanently basis.

Because these serious side effects occasionally occur, a man usually takes his first dose of Erectile Dysfunction medications under observation in a doctor's office. Doctors suggest taking the first dose of dysfunction medication under the supervision, due to the range of side effects and the potential for priapism.

Because of priapism (and the potential for scars), some men are unwilling to use injections as a way of gaining an erection.

Over the Counter (OTC) Treatments

Constriction and Vacuum Devices

Erections can be assisted by the use of a constriction device or a vacuum device, both of which are available over the counter. Economical and void of the damaging side effects other treatments can bring the major downfall of the devices are the bruising that can develop after use. They should not be used by men taking blood-thinning medication and should not be left on for longer than 30 minutes.

Constriction devices are commonly bands or rings made of rubber, metal or leather and are placed at the base of the penis to slow the outflow of blood. Alternatives in the market exist, with more extensive versions of these available to be purchased with a prescription and novelty versions purchased in sex stores (usually referred to as 'cock rings').

The devices are most effective in those with mild erectile dysfunction and those that struggle to maintain rather than gain an erection. They can be safely used with a vacuum device and rarely cause pain or interferes with ejaculation.

Vacuum devices (which consist of a hollow chamber attached to a source of suction) create a seal over the business. When suction is applied it immediately draws blood into the penis, producing an erection. Once an erection is achieved, a binding device is applied to prevent the blood from flowing out of the penis.

SURGICAL TREATMENT

If treatment in the methods already described is unsuccessful one option is to surgically attach prosthesis to help with erections.

A variety of suitable devices are available which range from a firm rod that is inserted into the penis (essentially a permanent erection) to the attachment of an inflatable balloon with a small pump. Both of the measures require a hospital stay and both will render the patient incapable of having intercourse for roughly 6 weeks.

Therapeutic Techniques

Psychological Therapy

Because psychological factors often compound the detrimental physical causes of impotence, some forms of psychological therapy (which include behavior-modification techniques, such as the sensate focus technique) can help to eradicate the internal demons preventing men achieving an erection. Generally speaking these can also help with the overall wellbeing and positivity of a sufferer.

Therapies are chosen based on the problems affecting the individual struggling with erectile dysfunction. For instance if the cause is depression, anti-depressants may work better than any other medication specifically for erectile dysfunction. Psychological treatments are as important as physical methods because they often have long-term appeal or benefits outside of sexual intercourse. For example, sometimes psychotherapy can reduce anxiety about sexual performance in which erectile dysfunction results, which in turn can create a more fulfilling relationship. This method is not a short term solution and requires a highly motivated and willing individual for psychotherapy to work.

Sex Therapy: The Sensate Focus Technique

One such psychotherapy technique that helps men with psychological sexual performance issues is called the sensate focus technique. It aims to open the channels of communicating between partners, so that both understand the sexual qualities they find pleasurable. This reduces performance anxiety and helps with the treatment of decreased libido, sexual arousal disorder, orgasmic disorder and erectile dysfunction (impotence).

Because this technique requires the attention of both parties, it is important both are comfortable with the level of detail discussed in sessions.

Step one is an intimate touching technique consisting of one partner's freedom to touch any other part of the others body excluding the genitals. The aim is to focus on the sensation of touching and not sexual arousal.

Secondly, the partners are then allowed to touch genitals with the focus remaining on touch not sexual sensation and no sexual intercourse is allowed.

The third and final step involves mutual touching, which this time can lead to sexual intercourse as the couple becomes more comfortable with each other and being touched. The focus is on comfort and enjoyment rather than on orgasm, effectively reducing a key source of performance anxiety.

Alternative Treatments and Natural Remedies

Having suggested that impotence can be formed by both psychical and psychological causes the following section will refute the claims favoring the mind as the greatest cause of impotence. An estimated 15 million American men are consistently unable to achieve or maintain erections, which points to physical causes as the reason not psychological factors.

In most cases, impotence can be attributed to a high-fat diet that can block the blood flow that causes erections. A lack of exercise or other reasons such as the wrong medication can leave men unaware of the impact small changes in their lives can have on their impotence. The natural remedies in this section, in conjunction with sound medical advice can go some way in relieving impotence.

You Need to See Your Medical Doctor

If you have diabetes or arteriosclerosis and aren't able to maintain an erection as frequently as usual; and your impotence is persistent or getting worse.

Acupressure:

"Acupressure on the Sea of Vitality points, B23 and B47, can fortify the body and, with repeated usage over a long period of time, can make a man stronger sexually," says Michael Reed Gach, Ph.D., Director of the Acupressure Institute in Berkeley, California, and author of Acupressure's Potent Points.

To find the B47 points, measure four finger widths away from the spine at the waist level. The points are situated on the lower back on the left and right sides of the spine, in line with the navel. From B47, you can move two finger widths closer to the spine to find the B23 points. Acupressurists believe that this pressure at points can help relieve pain and assist in sexual performance by alleviating dysfunction.

Dr. Gach says, "you can use your thumbs or fingers to work the points, pressing one or both B47 points for one minute, then one or both B23 points for one minute." He recommends using "this remedy three times daily adding that if you have a weak back press these points lightly, and be sure not to press directly on the disk or vertebrae."

Aromatherapy:

"Jasmine is often inhaled for its aphrodisiac qualities," writes San Francisco herbalist Jeanne Rose, Chairperson of the National Association for Holistic Aromatherapy, in her book, *Aromatherapy: Applications and Inhalations.* Because the oil is expensive, Rose suggests using it in a candle diffuser to make it last longer. It can also be inhaled from a handkerchief or applied directly to the body, she says.

As is often the case with effective treatments (especially in sensitive regions) people often expect Aromatherapy to hurt, however the treatments are in actual fact, often as simple as soothing lavender-scented baths an hot peppermint tea.

This is the basis of aromatherapy. These fragrant, pleasurable treatments are typical and represent a system of caring for the body with botanical oils. Oils can be added to a bath, massaged directly onto the skin, inhaled or diffused. Steeped in tradition, the natural oils have been used for nearly a thousand years to relieve pain, care for the skin, alleviate tension and fatigue and invigorate the entire body.

Aromatherapy has proven to be a popular home remedy and is becoming increasingly prevalent in major retailers such as Estée Lauder and the Body Shop who are selling the products like never before.

This is partly due to the increased awareness place on one's health and the wide range of publications and shows that support health, wealth and freedom. Most of today's generation look for ways to help themselves naturally and without side effects, therefore they should and often do consider aromatherapy.

How Aromatherapy Works

Aromatherapy works, mainly as the name suggests, by stimulating the sense of smell (a surprising powerful sense).

Aromatherapists have always believed in the powerful qualities in the oils used in their trade, but the practice is now getting more support from traditional medical avenues. Neurologist, psychiatrist and Director of the Smell and Taste Treatment and Research Center in Chicago, Dr. Alan Hirsch, M.D., says, "smells act directly on the brain, like a drug."

He goes on to say, "we know from brain wave frequency studies that smelling lavender increases alpha waves in the back of the head, which are associated with relaxation... An odor such as jasmine increases beta waves in the front of the head, which are associated with a more alert state."

Paraphernalia such as lamps, porcelain or clay pots, candles or diffusers are all available to extract the healing power of the essential oils and release them into a room, and thus the nose.

Aromatherapy experts are trained to assess how essential oils should be used. For instance some should not be used for certain conditions and others should not be used internally. Consult a specialist if you're unsure in this area.

Using Aromatherapy

Essential oils are on the cheaper scale of treatment options and are handy to have around the home for all purposes. They vary in price from $7 to $15 for a half-ounce vial of lavender oil, depending on its purity and where it's produced.

These are often highly concentrated and can last a long time due to only needing a small amount each use.

It is recommended that lavender oil is stored in glass or hard plastic bottles and kept in a cool, dark place. If you're contemplating buying some, most stores or mail-order companies that sell essential oils usually sell bottles as well.

Aromatherapy Cautions

Although much less likely to cause side effects than over the counter solutions for impotence, it's still vitally important to research and follow instructions for use carefully. As a precaution some fair skinned people with freckles are more likely to experience skin irritation from the use of essential oils.

Aromatic consultant, John Steele, advises all first-time users to perform a simple skin test to avoid allergic reactions. To perform a skin test, place a drop of the oil on a cotton swab and apply it to the inside of the wrist or to the inner elbow. Cover with a bandage and don't wash the area for 24 hours. If no itching or redness occurs, the oil should be safe for external use.

Ayurveda:

Here's a treatment regimen recommended by Vasant Lad, B.A.M.S., M.S.Sc., Director of the Ayurvedic Institute in Albuquerque, New Mexico, mix one cup of fresh grape juice with one teaspoon of fresh onion juice and a teaspoon of honey.

Drink this mixture daily, one hour before going to bed, for 45 days. Dr. Lad says it will help increase sexual energy and sperm count.

A core idea of Ayurveda is that the fundamental energy of life expresses itself through the three doshas; vata, pitta and kapha. Each person has a different mixture of doshas; usually, one dosha is predominant, and another is secondary. Ayurveda says that one of the main ways to keep your doshas balanced is through diet. If you don't eat according to your specific dosha, you will create an imbalanced state of the doshas.

"Men with kapha constitutions should add a pinch of trikatu," says Dr. Lad. Kaphas are sensuous, strong, calm, soft-spoken and forgiving. They tend to have well developed bodies with big but not prominent bones. Hair is plentiful, usually dark and wavy or curly. Kaphas frequently have oily complexions and large soulful eyes. Of all of the doshas, kaphas have the most trouble with their weight proportionate. Vatta people are creative, quick-witted and resourceful. Associated with the elements of space and air, vatas are active and alert and enjoy being on the move. Vatas can be quite softhearted and romantic. Pitta people are fiery, determined, strong-willed and passionate. They are tough-minded, clearheaded, enthusiastic and ambitious and can be quite successful. Pittas work well under pressure and can be courageous in emergencies. Out of balance, the pitta temper can be scary.

Dr. Lad explains that trikatu is an Indian herbal preparation combining dried ginger, black pepper, and pippali are available from Ayurvedic practitioners and by mail order. You can also purchase trikatu in some health food stores.

Please do not use this information to diagnose yourself or anyone else. It is always recommended to consult a certified expert in the field before implementing any of these techniques.

How to Find an Ayurvedic Practitioner

According to Dr. Lad, there are very few properly trained Ayurvedic practitioners in the United States. But there has been growing interest in both the philosophy of Ayurveda and in the practical details of Ayurvedic self-care.

There is however no licensing procedure and no accrediting board for Ayurvedic practitioners in the United States. Courses in Ayurveda are offered at various centers in the US, Canada, and Europe, but in the United States, graduates can only consult with clients, not practice medicine.

"If you interested in exploring Ayurvedic therapies, choose a practitioner who combines Western medical training with Ayurvedic training or coordinate Ayurvedic consultations with your regular M.D.," suggests Scott Gerson, M.D., an internist in New York City who has studied Ayurveda in India and is an Ayurvedic consultant.

According to Dr. Gerson, "Modern Western medicine works best when surgery or some other acute intervention is necessary. Ayurveda may serve better for the treatment of some chronic conditions and as preventive medicine." Experts suggest that this is because Ayurveda treats the causes of health problems, not the symptoms. Ayurveda can provide simple, effective treatment for chronic problems such as dizziness, fatigue, digestive complaints, tension headaches, and erectile dysfunction—problems that tend to frustrate Western medicine.

Ayurveda Daily Routine

If you're not in the care of an Ayurvedic practitioner but would like to try out Ayurveda's health care philosophy, you can start with some simple lifestyle adjustments that are part of the optimal Ayurvedic routine.

- Some of these include:
- Rising early (by 6am if possible);

- Meditating for at least 20 minutes once or twice each day;

Keeping your diet simple. A vegetarian or modified vegetarian diet is best. Make lunch a major meal of the day and eat a light dinner early in the evening, preferably between 5 and 6pm.

Ayurvedic treatments are usually simple involving lifestyle changes that can be made at once or over a period of time. Most Westerners find it hard to invest the necessary personal responsibility for changing a lifestyle that causes disease.

Two common Ayurveda treatments are:

Tribulus Terrestris is a natural treatment for erectile dysfunction. Rooted in Indian culture, Tribulus Terrestris is an Ayurveda practice that has been used as a tonic and aphrodisiac. Its Sanskrit name, for the flowering plant, is gokshura. It is being promoted as a testosterone booster used for the purpose of building muscle and increasing the sex drive.

Another interesting Ayurveda remedy that can be considered is mucuna pruriens, also known as 'velvet bean'. It is a climbing shrub with long vines that reach over 15m. Mucuna increases tissue resiliency and improves coordination. It can also support healthy testosterone levels, which in turn can lead to increase muscle mass and strength.

Flower Remedy / Essence Therapy

"If a visit to your doctor has ruled out physical causes of impotence, it may have an emotional cause," says Cynthia Mervis Watson, M.D., a family physician in Santa Monica, California, who specializes in homeopathic and herbal therapies. If a lack of sexual self-confidence is hampering you, Dr. Watson recommends the essence of Pink Monkey Flower. "If you're haunted by past episodes of impotence, the essence of Pink Monkey Flower may be helpful," she says.

"Impotence is always traumatic for a man, whether it's caused by physical or emotional factors," according to Dr. Watson. She says men receiving medical treatment for physically caused impotence can take the Bach flower remedy Star-of-Bethlehem, which will help them keep balanced emotionally. Flower remedies/essences are available in some health food stores and through mail order.

How Flower Remedy / Essence Therapy Works

Flower essences are the blossoms of plants prepared from a sun infusion in a bowl of water, then further diluted, potentized, and then preserved with brandy. Based on theories of balance and chi, flower essences are another great way to stimulate senses.

In history, flowers were nature's gentle tools for treating and preventing disease and practitioners have leapt on the traditional phenomenon to treat a range of modern illnesses.

"Many people are uncomfortable with the idea that their attitudes and emotions create health problems, because it makes them feel as if their illness were their fault," says Lynda Hammer, M.D., an Ayurvedic practitioner in Leavenworth, Washington, who uses the 38 flower remedies.

Co-director of the Flower Essence Society, Patricia Kaminski, says, "It's not enough to recognize your physical symptoms; you have to get to know yourself on a deeper level."

The success of flower remedies/essence therapy is still not entirely explainable, but researches suggest, much like aromatherapy and lavender the response stimulates the brain to release neurochemicals that alter emotions such as fear, anger and anxiety. In summary, the result is a strengthening of the body's innate ability to heal itself.

In addition to the 38 Bach remedies (The founder of Bach remedies is Dr. Edward Bach, an English physician), there are some practitioners who use the essences of flower species native to California. Many of them are Native American cures. These essences are distilled in a similar manner to Dr. Bach's method and are prescribed based on the mental and emotional state of the patient.

Flower essence is available to purchase from health food stores and from the manufacturers directly. They are all sold in concentrated form, so a little goes a long way. The most common form of intake is in water (one-fourth of a glass of water and sipped at intervals, usually first thing in the morning, before meals, and at bedtime). Since only a few drops of the remedy or essence is needed, a 10.5 milliliter bottle can last three to six months depending on use, and retails for about $8 to $9). Six remedies can be used at a time, but it is better practice to use only one at a time.

Once more, the reaction to flower essence remedies is not immediate. Patients will need to display patience and allow their bodies to adjust to the remedies and gradually shift the emotional difficulty. Herbalist Leslie Kaslof emphasizes, "The remedies aren't quick fixes." He also cautions that for those conditions or symptoms requiring medical attention, or if symptoms persist, a qualified health professional should be consulted.

Food Therapy

"You need to keep the arteries to the genitals open, and the way to do that is with a low- fat, low-cholesterol diet," says Michael A. Klaper, M.D., a nutritional medicine specialist in Pompano Beach, Florida, and director of the Institute of Nutrition Education and Research, an organization based in Manhattan Beach, California, that teaches doctors about nutrition and its relationship to disease. "That means a diet centered on plenty of high-fiber fresh fruits and vegetables, legumes and other low-fat fare," says Dr. Klaper.

Herbal Therapy

Ginkgo

"Supplements of the herb ginkgo, found in most health food stores, can improve blood flow to the penile arteries and veins, which may help reverse impotence," says herbalist James Green, Director of the California School of Herbal Studies in Forestville. He also warns that this herbal remedy isn't a quick fix; you'll need to take the supplements daily for six to eight weeks before you see results. Green says to follow dosage recommendations on the product label.

Existing research suggests that 1 of 60 men with impotence due to poor blood circulation demonstrated a 50 percent success rate after using it for six months. Further research dictates that ginkgo may be useful for impotence caused by drugs in the Prozac family as well as other types of medication that treat depression.

Although gingko is considered safe, it should not be mixed with blood- thinning drugs such as Coumadin (warfarin), heparin, aspirin, and Trental (pentoxifylline). If these chemicals are combined, bleeding problems may occur. Natural blood thinners, such as garlic, phosphatidylserine, and high doses of vitamin E, should not be combined with ginkgo.

Significant and dangerous side effects have occurred in the past, and reported cases include subdural hematomas, bleeding in the skull, and hyphema, bleeding into the iris chamber, with the use of gingko.

L-Arginine

An amino acid found in foods such as meat, dairy products, poultry and fish. The human body uses arginine to create nitric oxide, which in turn relaxing the blood vessels, and hopefully have a positive effect on symptoms of erectile dysfunction.

L-Arginine Caution

Although safe in moderate doses, around 2-3g per day, Arginine can provide minor digestive discomfort to those that take it. Not only that, but when the human body is exposed to high doses of arginine, it may cause the body to produce gastrin, a hormone that increases stomach acid. Accordingly, L-Arginine is not recommended for those with ulcers and people currently taking medication that upsets their stomach (e.g. liver disease).

Specifically, in relation to impotence, L-Arginine studies showed subjects experienced improvement in their sexual performance after just 6 weeks.

Zinc

Zinc is an element we only hear about when we have a deficiency, but many of us suffer from it, and it can cause impact sexual activity negatively.

In patients suffering from impotence, the common dose is 15-30mg daily, which should be supplemented with copper to reduce the chance of the zinc interfering with the bodies ability to absorb copper.

Zinc Caution

Too much zinc is toxic to the human body, so always keep to recommended doses.

Indian Ginseng (Ashwagandha)

Indian Ginseng is mainly used as a tonic herb and is capable of strengthening the entire body that includes sexual capacity. In short, many believe that Indian ginseng (which is not botanically related to Ginseng) is an aphrodisiac.

Helpful for those suffering from anxiety it can cause drowsiness so patients are warned not to take the favorite of holistic healers with other sedating drugs.

Natural Medicines

Traditional medicine is often the first port of call in western societies, due to our lack of understanding of alternatives, and due to our general upbringing of care and safety when it comes to health. Conventional medicine is also known as allopathic medicine and uses pharmaceutical and synthetic medicines manufactured and marketed according to societal norms and at the discretion of major corporations.

On the other side of allopathic medicine, comes homeopathic and herbal natural medicines which are becoming increasingly common more freely used. No medical assessment and treatment plan should be completed without consideration for both fields of medicine, as both have a part to play in nursing a patient back to health.

Evidence of the uptake of natural medicine by medical industry can be seen in the fact that medical schools now recognizing and offering tutelage of it in some of their courses. A doctor should be equipped with all the necessary tools to counteract an illness, especially when sexual gratification is at stake and so, natural medicine must be included in that tool kit.

In many countries, especially in Europe, India and China, natural and homeopathic medicines are commonly prescribed by conventional doctors and represent a significant part of the total annual drug sales.

Naturopathy is a branch of medicine (just as allopathy is too) that tries to teach the body its best qualities in a natural response to heal itself. Natural medicines are often harshly described as alternative or complimentary whereas they should be considered medicines in their own right, as they are able to treat conditions independently of traditional medicine. The better term is 'holistic' as it portrays the broad range of treatment options and approaches, which are to be found within the practice of natural medicine. Holistic medicines include herbalism, homeopathy, iridology, osteopathy, chiropractic, therapeutic massage techniques, aromatherapy, acupuncture and many, many more. A good naturopath will use all of the above treatment options to support the body's general health and wellness and help prevent disease and dysfunction.

The World Health Organization defines health as being "... more than simply the absence of illness. It is the active state of physical, emotional, mental and social well-being." The description is accurate in proving that holistic or natural medicine strives to support health (thereby relieving and preventing symptoms), rather than only eliminating disease.

While accepting the tremendous role allopathic medicine plays in the community it must be said that holistic medicine can reach the same heights. Medical science continues to develop as a subject and the contribution holistic medicine can make is endless. All without the risk of the side effects and addictions often plagued with traditional medicine.

As previously alluded to, holistic medicines can promote natural healing in an expeditious manner despite the negative publicity that often surrounds them. In fact, they can often work where pharmaceutical drugs have failed. As the exposure of the area of medicine improves, so to does the research dedicated to confirming its importance. They are now more widely researched by the major medical institutions and journals that are relevant in today's World.

Much like pharmaceutical drugs, holistic medicines are subject to rigorous testing and manufacturing guidelines. Acceptable procedures must be followed to ensure maximum effectiveness and safety. Those challenging demand shave not deterred the influx of companies now taking residence in the congested market. However the industry needs to be careful not to sour the name of holistic therapies by allowing inferior imitators in the market. Even big players in the pharmaceutical game have followed others to quickly produce their herbal range to fill the demand for natural medicine options.

The major companies do however produce product that have grave disadvantages from that of more authentic options. These include an increase in side effects as the natural protective qualities of the herbs are diminished in the rigid manufacturing process. In some cases, these side effects have proved fatal, for instance a case involving liver toxicity associated with standardized extracts of kava kava, an herb previously safely used for generations without any issues.

Differing from the heavily manufactured and standardized major company varieties, the herbal medicines retain the benefits of all the active ingredients with the assistance the full spectrum method of extraction. This provides a more complete treatment as well as superior protection against side effects.

This report recommends that you consider all and research all options that are available to combat your symptoms. It's also recommended that in doing so you speak to your doctor to ascertain the best course of action relevant to you. Most doctors will be open to discussing holistic remedies and will be encouraged by your willingness to take responsibility for your own health.

In the treatment of erectile dysfunction, the following herbal and homeopathic remedies are often used as part of the treatment plan.

Ikawe for Men

In response to the need to requests for an approach to erectile dysfunction without side effects, Native Remedies has developed Ikawe for Men - a 100% herbal remedy containing well researched ingredients, which is manufactured in therapeutic dosage according to the highest pharmaceutical standards.

Ikawe (which means 'Warrior" or "Strong") is a specially formulated all herbal formula containing selected phytoceutricals and adaptogens to optimize male sexual functioning, boost sexual performance and counteract the effects of modern living, drugs and environmental pollution.

Ikawe is a liquid tincture that contains selected phytoceutricals and adaptogens to promote normal, strong and healthy male sexual functioning. It helps maintain healthy functioning of the male reproductive system, along with balanced flow of blood to the penis and testes. Ikawe can make all the difference, without compromising health or risking serious side effects.

Use Ikawe To:
- Improve male sexual functioning
- Prevent Erectile Dysfunction and achieve strong, healthy erections
- Increase erect penis size
- Boost arousal and desire
- Raise sexual energy levels
- Achieve stronger and more pleasurable ejaculation
- Rejuvenate the male reproductive and hormonal systems
- Alleviate anxiety caused by problems in sexual performance

Ikawe contains the following therapeutic herbs in convenient and fast-acting drop format:

Epimedium grandiflorum, also known as Horny Goats Weed, is believed to help promote sexual desire and has been regarded for years in China and Japan as a 'natural sexual stimulator'! It is believed to promote healthy seminal emissions and encourage systemic harmony of the prostate gland and seminal vesicles. Epimedium species have long been used as sexual tonics in Chinese herbal medicine to encourage sexual performance and healthy testosterone production thus promoting sexual energy, and overall well-being. (Fukai T, Nomura T. "Seven prenylated flavonol glycosides from two Epimedium species". Phytochemistry. 1998;27:259-266). (Kessenich CR, Cichon MJ. "Hormonal decline in elderly men and male menopause". Geriatric Nursing. 2001; 22:24-28.)

Tribulus terristis has been studied for its ability to promote muscle health and strength and general prowess in the male body. (Rogerson S, Riches CJ, Jennings C, Weatherby RP, Meir RA, Marshall-Gradisnik SM. Abstract "The effect of five weeks of Tribulus terrestris supplementation on muscle strength and body composition during preseason training in elite rugby league players". J Strength Cond Res. 2007 May; 21(2):348-53. PMID: 17530942).

Animal studies have investigated the supporting effect of an extract of this herb on sexual desire. (Gauthaman K, Adaikan PG, Prasad RN. Abstract "Aphrodisiac properties of Tribulus Terrestris extract (Protodioscin) in normal and castrated rats". Life Sci. 2002 Aug 9;71(12):1385-96. PMID: 12127159).

Eleutherococcus senticosis, also known as Siberian ginseng, is one of the most important active ingredients in Siberian or Oriental Ginseng is the ginsenosides, which greatly promote healthy blood flow to the brain and peripherals, including the penis. In oriental medicine, Ginseng is highly respected and prized as a herb which promotes male or 'yang' energy, aiding circulation, supporting natural vitality and acting as an overall systemic supporter.

It can combat stress and is a supportive tonic for healthy adrenal hormones. In a recent study Siberian ginseng was shown to support stamina and fitness. (Szolomicki J, Samochowiec L, Wojcicki J, Drozdzik M, Szolomicki S. "The influence of active components of Eleutherococcus senticosus on cellular defence and physical fitness in man". Phytother Res. 2000 Feb; 14(1): 30-5). (Hartz AJ, Bentler S, Noyes R, et al. "Randomized controlled trial of Siberian ginseng for chronic fatigue". Psychol Med . 2004;34(1):51-61).

In addition, animal studies lend growing support for the use of ginseng in lessening sexual dysfunction and studies provide increasing evidence for a role of ginsenoside action utilizing nitric oxide. [The effects of ginseng on the corpus cavernosum (one of two parallel columns of erectile tissue forming the dorsal part of the body of the penis) appear to be mediated by the release and/or modification of release of nitric oxide from endothelial cells and perivascular nerves]. (Murphy LL, Lee TJ. "Ginseng, sex behavior, and nitric oxide". Department of Physiology, Southern Illinois University, School of Medicine, Carbondale, Illinois 62901, USA. 2002 May; 962:372-7 PMID: 12076988).

Sabal serrulata, also known as Saw Palmetto, has long been utilized by the Seminole Indians as a tonic to promote strength. Extracts from the fruit of this short, scrubby palm have been used historically to address urogenital health. Many modern clinical trials corroborate the ability of saw palmetto extract (SPE) to lessen the signs and symptoms of prostate conditions, for which it is a first-line treatment in much of Europe. (Buck A. Phytotherapy for the prostate. Br J Urol. 1996; 78:325-336). (Lowe F, Ku J. Phytotherapy in treatment of BPH: a critical review. Urology. 1996; 48:12-20). Saw palmetto enhances the actions of other herbs - thus, it helps support the prostate gland's healthy hormone balance necessary for optimal sexual function. (Murray, M, "Extract of serenoa repens in the treatment of benign prostatic hyperplasia", Phyto-Pharmica Review, vol 1, p. 5, August 1988).

Smilax ornate, also known as Sarsaparilla, contains steroidal saparins which are thought to mimic the action of some human hormones. It is used as a supportive tonic to the male reproductive system and is thought to promote healthy routine production of testosterone and progesterone.

Glycorrhyza glabra, also known as Liquorice, originates in the Mediterranean and the Middle East and has many uses, including being a supportive tonic for the adrenal cortex. It promotes the natural production of hormones such as hydrocortisone that has steroidal anti-inflammatory agents.

Kola vera, also known as Kola nut, has active constituents of this herb which include tannins, proteins, additional phenolics and anthrocyanin (that are likely to provide antioxidant activity). In addition, Kola vera contains a unique constellation of Xanthines that are regarded as utilized elements to lessen common fatigue and support the body's natural ability to rejuvenate and replenish it's routine energy levels.

Epimedium Grandiflorum extract is also commonly known as 'horny goat weed'. It has been over 2000 years since horny goat weed has been used in reproductive beverages for boosting the sex drive and treating erectile dysfunction.

As high stress cause fatigue and lessens sexual desire, substitutes (or aphrodisiacs) are sought to improve energy and thus sex drive. This herb and horny goat weed are well established such substitutes. Studies report this herb as being a time tested aphrodisiac due to its restoration of testosterone and thyroid.

Unsurprisingly, an active ingredient in goat weed(e.g. a flavonoid, among others, called icarin) is also found in prescription drugs such as Viagra, Cialis, and Levitra.

A men's sexual supplement called Vuka Nkuzi contains Lepidium Meyenii, which is also known as Maca Root and provides a wide range of medicinal benefits. Mainly in infertility, erectile dysfunction, and sexual activity issues.

Homeopathy

"After a thorough medical examination and diagnosis, try taking one of these remedies two or three times a day until improvement occurs," says Chris Meletis, N.D., a naturopathic physician and Medicinary Director at the National College of Naturopathic Medicine in Portland, Oregon.

Agnus castus can be helpful for symptoms of a cold and relaxed penis and for lack of sexual desire, especially if accompanies by a fear of death and dilated pupils, says Dr. Meletis. If you are apprehensive and cannot have an erection or if erections lead to premature ejaculation, Dr. Meletis recommends Lycopodium. "Try Argentum nitricum, if your erection fails when attempting intercourse, if intercourse is painful and if your symptoms are made worse at night, from warmth and when you eat sweets." All of these remedies are available in health food stores.

Imagery

"Conquering impotence may be as simple as conquering an ogre," writes Gerald Epstein, M.D., a New York City psychiatrist and author of Healing Visualizations. Here's an example provide by Dr Epstein on how this can work.

Imagine yourself descending into a valley. Where a monster or an ogre confronts you. Fortunately, you have everything you need to defeat this beast. Fight the monster, and when you are triumphant and the monster is dead, skin it. Carry the skin with you and climb to the top of the valley. There you meet your loved one. Take her hand, walk with her to a tree and lie behind it. Picture the two of you surrounded by a cocoon of blue light and embrace.

Dr Epstein suggests practicing this technique for five to seven minutes once a week, on the same morning each week, for three weeks.

Reflexology

"Pay special attention to the diaphragm reflex as well as the spine, reproductive system and pituitary, parathyroid, thyroid and adrenal gland reflexes on your feet," says reflexologist Dwight Byers, author of Better Health with Foot Reflexology.

How to Work the Points

According to Mr. Byers, Reflexology is a complex, thorough system. Reflexology is not the same as just rubbing your feet all over. The idea is that pressure applied to the feet and hands promote a beneficial response throughout the body, providing a break from stress.

The feet provide strong clues as to the balance of the entire body according to professional reflexologist, and they'll often use the feet to assess any given patients situation. For example, a tender spot on the feet could demonstrate a problem in the corresponding part of the body.

Not that reflexologists are able to diagnose or help in the treatment of their findings. They predominantly focus on the sore spots of the feet only.

That is why professional reflexologists insist that their work is best suited for prevention. Prevention benefits include better blood circulation, which results in the clearing out of impurities, effectively balancing your system, and giving you more energy.

Your Reflexology Session

Anyone can try reflexology in his or her own home. All you need is a few thumb and finger techniques and a guide map and you can start immediately. The basics of reflexology are very easy to pick up. Here are some tips:

The thumb walk is the most common technique.

You use the outside edge of your thumb to take small "bites" of the hand or foot, applying gently, steady pressure as you go. The finger walk is similar to the thumb walk, except that you use the edge of your index finger to take the bites on the hands or foot. The hook and back up technique puts steady pressure on a single point. You place your thumb on the reflex point, then pull back slightly to "grab" the point. Rotation on a point also puts pressure on a single point and is better to use when you encounter a tender area. Additionally, a golf ball may be used to apply pressure to small points, usually on the hand.

Reflexology's foundation is built on pressure.

The technique above depends on the sixe of the area and how much pressure is needed to apply the treatment directly. Much like gym routine or a yoga session, reflexology can be added to a daily exercise and wellness regime.

Sessions should average approximately 30 minutes each, especially if you're dealing with a problem area.

Starting with relaxation techniques such as pressing between the toes, across the soles and over the tops of the feet, or on your hands, pressing between the fingers and cross the palms will work to loosen the areas.

Moving into the actual treatment, the starting point is at the top of the left foot, and then working down the foot as pressure is applied to tender spots and to specific areas. Afterwards, work your foot a second time continuing to apply pressure to tender spots and specific areas. At each spot, press firmly to the point where it each spot hurts but also feels relieving. Repeat on the right foot and hands.

The sensation of 'good pain' cannot be confused with bruising and it is important not to apply pressure too hard. For instance, if an area of the hand or foot is bony, pressure should be lighter, whilst fleshier areas can withstand more pressure.

Relaxation and Meditation

Biofeedback:

Relaxation and mediation can also aid in the relief of a number of conditions and is worth considering in improving sexual experience. Biofeedback for instance aids in the relief of varied conditions, not just impotence, these include muscle spasms, tooth grinding and epilepsy. Professionals in the mental health sector also believe the biofeedback works well in conjunction with other relaxation techniques.

The biofeedback process involves attaching electrodes to the body whereby the electrodes monitor and report back on the body's functions. Changes in any of these electrodes can be detected instantly by the biofeedback machine and provided to the professional in control of the machine. The best way to use this feedback is to regulate bodily functions based on the results so that you feel more relaxed.

Thermal Biofeedback at Home

An easier (and cheaper) method than the professional version above involves thermal biofeedback in your own home. Simply using a thermometer and your hands, the process takes just 15 minutes.

"Daily practice of thermal biofeedback can often help overcome impotence because it reduces anxiety and keeps your blood vessels open," says Steven Fahrion, Ph.D., Director of Research at the Life Sciences Institute of Mind-Body and Health in Topeka, Kansas.

Dr. Fahrion says, "Many people haven't heard of it, although it has been used in hospitals and clinics to treat stress-related disorders such as high blood pressure for more than 20 years. Most people can learn to do it in a single session."

Thermal feedback was developed in the Menninger Clinic in Topeka, Kansas. According to this clinic, thermal biofeedback is based on the underlying premise that when a person is under stress, the hands and feet often reflect the restricted flow of blood associated with stress and therefore display the mindset readily. In the alternative, if you warm your hands, blood flow increases; stress hormones diminish; muscles relax; and you'll feel less tense.

To practice at home, relax in a comfortable position and wrap your hands around a thermometer so that your fingertips are touching. Resting your hands in your lap and focusing the mind on any sensation that you feel in your fingers, you should feel a tingling or pulsing in your fingertips, which is a sign that your hands are warming. Over time, your natural temperature should rise when your willing it to do so and your intention is to warm. It's important to focus for the entire time of the exercise.

Dollemore, Doug, et al., New Choices in Natural Healing, Pennsylvania: Rodale Press, Inc., 1995:

The principle behind relaxation and meditation is that peace of mind heals. Modern scientific evidence is only now proving the truth of this ancient therapeutic process. Dr. Fahrion says, "Relaxation and meditation can have a very powerful effect on the body. It can help you cope with all kinds of stress-related problems, including migraines, peptic ulcers, and anxiety. So I think that people who develop and retain peace of mind do experience mental and physical healing."

Studies imply that relaxation and mediation techniques can boost immunity, short- circuit anger, curb smoking and relieve insomnia, back pain, high blood pressure, motion sickness, impotence, menopause and irritable bowel syndrome. With the aid of professional assistance, these techniques can also help control diseases, such as diabetes, psoriasis, rheumatoid arthritis, panic attacks, phobias and depression.

As the major contributor to psychological disease, stress can impact affect almost every aspect of your body. Chronic stress, for instance, elevates blood pressure, total blood cholesterol, and blood platelet counts. All of these lead to atherosclerosis (hardening of the arteries) and heart attack. Research indicates that a staggering eight out of ten people seen by primary care physicians have a stress-related symptoms.

One way to counteract the effects of stress is to indulge in meditation and relaxation to give the mind an appropriate break. Relaxation is a physiological state that reduces muscles tension, lowers heart rates and blood pressure, and eases breathing which all add up to lessens feelings of stress. Eileen Stuart, R.N., Director of Cardiovascular Programs at the Mind-Body Medical Institute, a behavioral medicine clinic at Deaconess Hospital in Boston says that relaxation is the combination of the factors above leaving the mind in a tranquil place.

"The relaxation response blunts the release of adrenaline, catecholamines and other stress hormones that trigger the fight-or-flight response," Stuart says. This is important because an overdose of stress hormones can suppress the immune system and elevate blood cholesterol levels.

Dr. Fahrion says, "This type of deep relaxation is associated with healing in many different ways. When you get very deeply relaxed, for example, the body releases growth hormones that help repair and restore damaged tissue." Before you begin, however, please note that these techniques will not prevent stress from occasionally disrupting your life.

Five Relaxation Enhancers:

Relaxation and meditation techniques are a surprisingly strong response to stress and anxiety and can do wonders for the body and the mind. Five such processes, provided in New Choices in Natural Healing by Doug Dollemore, et al., are ideal for achieving inner peace and balance, they are:

1. **Stomp Out the Cigarettes and Cigars**:   Despite the large number of pitfalls and smoking (including cancers and heart disease) smoking also poses a risk to the stress hormone levels in the body. Hence, quitting is recommended to minimize the fluctuations in stress hormones and become more relaxed.

2. **Moderate the Caffeine:** Caffeine is a stimulant and can therefore affect the arousal and stress levels in the bodies. Like alcohol, drugs and cigarettes, the body can become depend on caffeine, which affects the stress balance. It is recommended we avoid coffee, tea and energy drinks.

3. **Limit the Carbs**: Even though health and nutrition experts will have us reduce carbs from a weight loss perspective, our advice asks you to commit to eating grains, vegetables and fruits loaded with complex carbohydrates. These carbohydrates trigger the release of hormones that will help you relax. It is important these are 'good carbohydrates' however such as sweet potato, whole-wheat pasta and beans.

4. **Generate a Sweat:** Common sense tells us that exercise plays an important part of the natural functioning of the human body. Thus a regular exercise regime will control anxiety and self-esteem. Thirty minutes of exercise a day is recommended.

5. **Commit to A Daily Chuckle:** A chemical in the brain called endorphins produces Euphoria. These endorphins suppress the feeling of stress and sadness and promote better self-esteem and happiness. One of the key ways to generate endorphins is through laughter, resulting in a more relaxing state.

"This type of deep relaxation is associated with healing in many different ways," Dr. Fahrion says. "When you get very deeply relaxed, for example, the physical body releases growth hormones that help repair and restore damaged tissue."

Vitamin and Mineral Therapy

"Vitamin A deficiency has been the cause of impotence in some men," says Elson Haas, M.D., Director of the Preventive Medical Center of Mann in San Rafael, California, and author of Staying Healthy with Nutrition. Although vitamin A can be toxic in large doses, Dr. Haas says that most men can safely take between 10,000 and 25,000 international units daily without dangerous side effects, but he recommends consulting a doctor before undertaking this supplementary option on your own.

Other nutrient compounds called phytochemicals have beneficial effects on health and are available in the hundreds. As an example, some researchers have attempted to ward off cancer with the use of these phytochemicals in vegetables.

Unfortunately our daily intakes of fruit and vegetables and the included chemicals mean we only get a minute amount of the beneficial compounds and thus need to supplement our diet to address the deficiency.

Richard Anderson, Ph.D., lead scientist for the nutrient requirements and functions laboratory at the U.S. Department of Agriculture Human Nutrient Research Center in Beltsville, Maryland, says, "There is overwhelming evidence that supplements have beneficial effects on a person's health, because they offer much higher doses of key nutrients than you find in food—sometimes amounts that you could never get from diet alone."

A Little History

Foods play an important part of in giving us the minerals and nutrients we need to boost our immunity and generally balance the body. That means, food has been used for centuries as therapy for common ailments. An example of the history surrounding the role food plays in health is in the ancient Egyptians belief that a lack of vitamin A caused night blindness. Hence, they ate the livers of roosters and oxen to cure night blindness, in conjunction with sea sponge as a natural source of iodine to treat goiters.

In 1906, research started to suggest that food only might not be enough to provide the support we needed in our daily lives and the isolation of the nutrient compounds in foods revealed that we needed 'vitamines' to supplement our diets; the e was dropped some years later.

Vitamins were then ranked alphabetically in the order they were discovered. The next section will provide a cross section of the vitamins that are now common in society because of the early research and developments. The table will also look at the recommended daily use of each and where to get it.

Getting What You Need

Nutrient	RDA	Daily Value	Benefits	Food Sources
Vitamin A	1,000mcg. RE or 5,000 IU	5,000 IU	Need for normal vision in dim light; maintains normal structure and function of mucous membranes; aids growth of bones, teeth and skin;	Carrots, pumpkin, sweet potatoes, spinach, butternut squash, tuna, cantaloupe, mangoes, apricots, broccoli, watermelon;
B Vitamins				
Thiamin	1.5 mg.	1.5 mg	Carbohydrate metabolism; maintains healthy nervous system;	Pork, wheat germ, pasta, peanuts, legumes, watermelon, organs, brown rice, oatmeal, eggs;
Riboflavin	1.7 mg	1.7 mg	Fat, protein and carbohydrate metabolism; health skin	Milk, cottage cheese, avocados, tangerines, prunes, asparagus, broccoli, mushrooms, beef, salmon, turkey;

Niacin	19 mg.	20 mg	Fat, protein and carbohydrate metabolism; nervous system function; needed for oxygen use by cells;	Meats, poultry, fish, peanut butter, legumes, soybeans, whole-grain cereals and breads, broccoli, asparagus, baked potatoes;
Vitamin B6	2.0 mg	2.0 mg	Protein metabolism; needed for normal growth;	Fish, soybeans, avocados, lima beans, chicken, bananas, cauliflower, green peppers potatoes, spinach, raisins;
Folate (folic acid)	200 mcg.	0.4 mg. (400 mcg.)	Red blood cell development; tissue growth and repair;	Legumes, poultry, tuna, wheat germ, mushrooms, oranges, asparagus, broccoli, spinach, bananas, strawberries, cantaloupe;
Vitamin B12	2.0 mcg.	6.0 mcg.	Needed for new tissue growth, red blood cells, nervous system and skin;	Salmon, eggs, cheese, swordfish, tuna, clams, crab, mussels, oysters.
Biotin	30-100 mcg. *	0.3 mg. (300 mcg.)	Fat, protein and carbohydrate metabolism	Peanut butter, eggs, oatmeal, wheat germ, poultry, cauliflower, nuts, legumes;
Pantothenic acid	4.7 mg. *	10 mg.	Fat, protein and carbohydrate metabolism;	Fish, whole-grain cereals, mushrooms, avocados, broccoli, peanuts, cashews, lentils, soybeans, eggs;
Vitamin C	60 mg.	60 mg.	Builds collagen; maintains healthy gums; teeth and blood vessels	Oranges, grapefruit, bell peppers, strawberries, tomatoes, spinach, cabbage, melons, broccoli, kiwifruit, raspberries;
Vitamin D	5 mcg.	400 IU (10 mcg.)	Calcium absorption; growth of bones and teeth	Sunlight, eggs, milk, butter, tuna, salmon, cereals, baked goods (if fortified flour is used)

Vitamin E	10 mg. Alpha- TE or 15 IU	30 IU	Protect cells from damage	Nut and vegetable oils, wheat germ, mangoes, blackberries, apples, broccoli, peanuts, spinach, whole wheat breads;
Vitamin K	80 mcg.	None	Blood clotting	Spinach, broccoli, Brussels sprouts, cabbage, parsley, eggs, dairy products, carrots, avocados, tomatoes;
Calcium	800 mg.	1 g. (1,000 mg.)	Strong bones and teeth; muscle and nerve function; blood clotting;	Milk, cheese, yogurt, salmon and sardines with bones, broccoli, green beans, almonds, turnip greens, fortified orange juice;
Chloride	750 mg.†	None	Aids digestion; works with sodium to maintain fluid balance;	Foods with salt;
Copper	1.5—3.0 mg. *	None	Strengthens tooth enamel	Fluoridated water, fish, tea
Iodine	150 mcg.	150 mcg.	Maintains proper thyroid function;	Spinach, lobster, shrimp, oysters, milk, iodized salt;
Magnesium	350 mg.	400 mg.	Aids nerve and muscle function; strong bones;	Molasses, nuts, spinach, wheat germ, pumpkin seeds, seafood, dairy products, baked potatoes, broccoli, bananas;
Manganese	2.0-5.0 mg. *	None	Bone and connective tissue formation; fat and carbohydrate metabolism;	Nuts, whole-grain cereals, legumes, tea, dried fruits, spinach and other green leafy vegetables;

Molybdenum	75-250 mcg. *	None	Nitrogen metabolism	Legumes, meats, whole-grain cereals, breads, milk and milk products;
Phosphorus	800 mg.	1 g. (1,000 mg.)	Energy metabolism; teams up with calcium for strong bones and teeth;	Meats, fish, poultry, eggs, dairy products, cereals;
Potassium	2,000 mg.†	3,500 mg.	Controls acid balance in the body; works with sodium to maintain fluid balance;	Baked potatoes, avocados, dried fruits, yogurt, cantaloupe, spinach, bananas, mushrooms, milk, tomatoes;
Selenium	70 mcg.	None	Helps vitamin E protect cells and body tissue;	Meats, whole-grain cereals, dairy products, fish, hellfish, mushrooms, Brazil nuts;
Sodium	500 mg.†	2.400 mg.	Fluid balance; nervous system function	Salt, processed foods, soy sauce, seasonings;
Zinc	15 mg.	15 mg.	Wound healing; growth; appetite; sperm production;	Oysters, lean beef, wheat germ, seafood, lima beans, legumes, nuts, poultry, dairy products;

* Value is the Estimated Safe and Adequate Daily Intake. There is no RDA for this nutrient

† Value is the estimated Minimum Requirement. There is no RDA for this Nutrient.

Reference: Dollemore, Doug, et al. New Choices in Natural Healing, Pennsylvania: Rodale Press, Inc., 1995

Vitamins are so good for us because they contain carbon, a substance found only in living things. This point illustrates the natural qualities of vitamins, which can sometimes be confused with minerals. Minerals, while good for the body, are non-organic compounds and consequently only found in smaller quantities in foods. Dr. Michael Janson, M.D., director of the Center of Preventive Medicine in Barnstable,

Massachusetts and an officer of the American College for Advancement in Medicine, says, "Along with essential fatty acids and amino acids, vitamins and minerals are among the almost 50 known essential nutrients we need for a healthy life."

Of the recommended vitamins fore everyday use, four of them (A, D, E and K) are fat-soluble, meaning that excess amounts can be stored in the body. Vitamin C and the eight B vitamins, are water-soluble, which is in contrast to the fat-soluble vitamins, water-soluble simply means and excess amounts in the body are passed out through urination.

Because minerals are contained in small amounts in each food source they are harder to identify and were discovered after vitamins. Minerals are classified into two categories: major minerals, or macronutrients, such as calcium, magnesium and potassium, found in relatively high concentrations in food; and trace minerals, or micronutrients, such chromium, copper, iron and zinc, found only in minuscule amounts.

Every single nutrient listed in the table earlier plays an important role in stabilizing the nervous and immunity systems. Whether taken in one's everyday diet via the food they eat or supplemented in a tablet or pill, they are the building blocks of the health of every organ in the body.

According to Dr. Janson, the most important fact to note about vitamins and minerals, is that every cell in your body needs every vitamin; however not every cell utilizes them in the same way or needs the same amounts. Because of that, it is hard to know for sure which vitamins or minerals are the most important in fighting disease (and for the purposes of this report sexual impotence).

Power Vitamins and Minerals

A Radical Response with Vitamins

For the maximum protection against common illness and for the best response to fighting a current ailment, the crème de la crème of vitamins (called antioxidants) should be taken. Essentially, these are vitamins C and E and beta-carotene, a form of vitamin A. When taken in the correct doses, this powerful trio can offer protection against 60 age- related afflictions, from cancer and cataracts to heart disease and high cholesterol.

How Do They Work?

The power vitamins work by stopping the toxic chemicals called free radicals. Free radicals are caused by radiation, cigarette smoke, car exhaust, and other pollutants cause free radicals, and eat away at healthy cells rendering them ineffective. The annoying response is the same way cancer cells spread through the body, and can eventually lead to changes to cholesterol levels, blockages in arteries, actual cancer and a general increase in the aging process.

How to Make It Benefit You the Most

As the body adjusts to taking different supplements the effects can change or diminish over time and it is therefore important to understand the different kinds of vitamins and minerals you'll need at different stages of your life. Because of the changes in the way the body absorbs vitamins, they become more important as you age.

Even the healthiest and active individuals can benefit from supplements. "Moderate exercise enhances immunity, but if you're running more than 30 miles a week or doing a lot of other type of exercise, you can actually hurt immunity and be more prone to viruses," says Kenneth H. Cooper, M.D., Founder and President of the Cooper Aerobics Center in

Dallas. His recommendation for those individuals who exercise a lot is to take vitamin supplements rich in antioxidants. The recommended dosage is 1,000 milligrams of vitamin C, 400 international units (IU) of vitamin E in the natural alpha-tocopherol form and 15 milligrams (25,000 IU) of beta-carotene each day.

The power antioxidants are dominating the attention in the media but many experts believe the developments in minerals will be equally as exciting. "There is a lot of exciting research being done with minerals right now," says Dr. Anderson.

The excitement and potential around minerals comes from the dosages that an individual cannot find through food alone. A good example of this is in the trace mineral, chromium. According to Dr. Anderson, chromium has been shown to reduce risk factors for diabetes and cardiovascular disease in some people. He says, "It improves glucose and insulin and lowers cholesterol and triglycerides, a form of blood fat that has been linked to an increased risk of heart disease. Give someone the recommended 50 micrograms, and he'll get along fine. But if you want protection against heart disease, you need 400 micrograms. And research shows that copper and magnesium can protect against heart disease—but only in amounts that you rarely get from food."

Zinc is proving a popular option for fighting off invading infections and keeping the immune system strong. In some cases it is proving more popular than antioxidants, and in fact, in addition to helping with impotence, it is a great option for the common cold. That's because they kill many of the germs that cause sore throats and other bacteria associated with the common cold.

The recommended daily intake (RDA) of zinc is set at 15 milligrams for men, which is more than most people currently get (somewhere between 8 and 10 milligrams). For this reason, Amanda Prasad, M.D. Ph.D., professor of medicine at Wayne State University in Detroit and a leading expert on zinc, says, "I'd say about 30 milligrams a day—more if they're having a specific skin problem or another condition."

As we discussed earlier in this chapter zinc will help with a rage of conditions but only if properly balanced with copper.

Rounding off the list of powerful minerals is Selenium. It has antioxidant qualities that protects against heart disease and cancer, alleviates symptoms of arthritis, and can even improve mood. Against an RDA of 70 micrograms for men, Dr. Janson recommends taking up to six times that amount each day to reap these rewards.

Victory with Vital Vitamins

Issues with impotence reinforce the importance of a strong immunity and a nutrient essential to a strong immunity is vitamin B6. Even more effective with old age the vitamin restores levels of B6 that are lost through the aging process. It is recommended that 50 to 100 milligrams of vitamin B6 be taken daily.

Summary

In conclusion, supplements help to create an overall package of health and wellbeing, and are not a stand-alone solution. Vitamins, minerals and antioxidants form only part of the solution to ailing health or protection against potential health concerns. When combined with professional medical advice, a sound exercise regime, a healthy diet and the limitation of cigarettes and alcohol, all patients young and old can reap the rewards of taking them.

Yoga

Yoga has played an important part in the relaxation strategies of enthusiasts for years but now a yoga pose called "the knee squeeze may fight against impotence," according to Alice

Christensen, Founder and Executive Director of the American Yoga Association. She recommends the combination of this exercise with two inverted yoga poses (the easy bridge and the cobra). Such a simple measure is easy to incorporate into a daily routine that recognizes the importance of breathing techniques and meditation. This can be done in one workout or during short sharp meditation breaks of ten minutes throughout a day.

The Knee Squeeze Pose

The pose credited for helping impotence is easy to perform. Lie face up on the floor or a mat. Your hands should be at your sides, and your toes should be slightly pointed. Inhale slowly and fully as you raise your right knee to your chest. Grab the knee with both arms and hold it to your chest for a few seconds. Then begin to exhale as you straighten your knee and lower it slowly to the floor. Repeat with the left leg. Do this a total of three times, alternating legs.

To match the pose, control your breathing with deep breaths, while bringing both knees to your chest at the same time. Wrap your arms around both legs and hold for a few seconds, then breathe out and lower your legs.

Those of us who are especially flexible can extend this stretch as much as they can, but please use caution if you experience pain or discomfort.

The Easy Bridge Pose

Lie on the floor or a mat. Your knees should be bent. Place your feet flat on the floor and as close to your buttocks as possible. Your hands should be at your sides, with palms down.

Breathe out slowly as you relax your head, neck and shoulders. As you start to breathe in, lift your hips off the floor slowly. Arch your back, with your shoulders and neck remaining on the floor. Hold this position for one or two breaths. Then slowly lower your hips to the floor as you exhale. Repeat two more times.

Cobra Pose

Lie facedown with your forehead touching the floor. Your toes should be pointed, with the tops of your toes touching the floor. Place your hands, palms down, on the floor next to your armpits.

Lift your head slowly off the floor as you begin to take a breath. Be sure to look straight up. Now lift your chest and stomach off the floor. Use the muscles of the back to lift, curling your spine.

Men should not attempt this pose if they have open wounds in the abdominal region or if they have undergone abdominal or pelvic surgery within the past several weeks.

Breathing Exercises

Daily yoga involves four succinct aspects; breathing, relaxation, meditation and poses. Together, they relax the body and distress the mind while relieving aches and pains and building flexibility and strength. All of which helps lift a weight of your shoulders and helps you find inner peace.

All yoga session should begin with concentrated breathing exercises, and last for approximately 30 minutes. Alice Christensen, founder and executive director of the American Yoga Association, reports that deep breaths deliver energy into your body; provides you with essential oxygen; and calms your muscles and organs.

Breathing exercises are important because we are naturally trained to take shorter breaths, particularly when exercising. Shallow breaths prevent our lungs from expanding enough to soak up enough oxygen to truly gain the benefits breathing exercises can bring. Much like signers are trained, the correct technique is using the diaphragm, which is the thin muscle underneath your lungs. When this thin muscle flexes, the lower lobes of your lungs are pulled down and opens. This process allows more air inside your lungs. Alice Christensen calls this type of breathing the belly breath. It was so named because your belly expands as air enters the lungs, not your chest.

In short, the belly breath involves sitting comfortably in a chair or on the floor with the hips tilt slightly forward. Then put one hand on your stomach and breathe out slowly through your nose, contracting your stomach muscles and lightly pushing on your stomach. When breathing in, relax your stomach muscles, arch your back slightly and let the air flow in your nose, and the result is a slight shift of your hand from your belly.

According to Christensen, this is the proper way to breathe all the time, delivering health gains in everyday life, breath by breath. "Chest breathing comes from stress; it's a reaction to stress. But breathing from the belly is a natural way to relax and spread more oxygen to your entire body."

Breathing techniques can be more extensive than the simple belly technique and yoga theory outlining how some can be used to clear the sinuses, some to strengthen stomach and chest muscles, and some to reduce stress. Experts say the latter reason, is why we should all practice breathing techniques for a few minutes each day as part of yoga routines.

The complete breath is a more extensive option than the belly breath and starts just like it. The difference is your hands are in a different position. Place them on either side of your lower rib cage, with your fingers touching slightly. Now, begin breathing from your stomach. Let the air fill your lower lungs. Then, let the breath begin to fill the lower part of your chest. Try to make your ribs expand sideways as your lungs fill. You should feel your fingers spreading apart as your chest expands.

Keep drawing in more air, working towards the top of your lungs. Straighten your shoulders and arch your back, letting the air completely fill up your lungs. As a caution, do remember not to breathe so deeply that you feel straining in your stomach or chest muscles.

The complete inhalation should last for ten seconds. The length of your exhalation should be the same. To help control your breath better, always breathe through your nose.

This type of deep breathing technique can also work at any time you're experiencing high stress.

Now for Your Mind...

The breathing techniques work on the body leaving an opportunity to also work on your mind. To do this, yoga instructors recommend you spend some time each day to think about absolutely nothing.

This is effectively known as mediation and it helps us focus on ourselves allowing us to discover more about us as people and our bodies as temples. Relaxation gently pulls you into mediation. According to yoga instructor Lilias Folan, "Meditation is something you do by yourself without children or pets in the room. No telephones. Eventually, you'll be able to stay centered and calm when there are distractions. And when you get off base, you'll know how to return to the center through the use of your breathing and relaxation techniques."

To try advanced meditation we suggest looking at the American Yoga Associations programs that guide and assist novices to try the technique using a position on your back called the corpse pose. The association's founder and executive director says this position allows you to relax completely, since there's no pressure on any of your limbs.

Corpse Pose

Lie on your back on either the floor or a mat. Your arms should be at your sides, with the palms of your hands facing up. Your legs should be straight, with your feet in a relaxed position. Relax all of your muscles, close your eyes and hold the pose for 30 seconds to several minutes, until your muscles completely relax. Breathe deeply and scan your body to feel any tension. If you feel tension, concentrate on the area and relax the muscles.

Considering Yoga?

A great place to start for yoga newbies is a group fitness class at your local health club or YMCA. These are great ways to learn the techniques of others and work at your own pace and development. Moreover they are cheap and varied so you can find one that suits your needs. If a group class is not in your interests, try a home video or internet/smartphone app that will teach you variety of posses and techniques.

Most classes teach hatha yoga, a traditional type using common poses and mediation, but the type of lesson will differ dramatically. One teacher might be more inclined to promote stretching rather than relaxation, as might another stress the importance of meditation rather than flexibility. Once again, the advice is to find something that work for you. Doing some is better than doing none.

Home Meditation

You don't need to find a yoga class or pay for a gym membership just to experience meditation (if you don't want to). Home techniques can work just as well and are easy to perform. Find a dimly lit, warm room with no drafts. Place a mat or blanket on the floor and lie on it face up. Do not use a pillow unless your doctor has advised you that you need to keep your head raised for medical reasons. Now spend about five minutes unwinding. Focus your mind on the different parts of your body. Concentrate on feeling them release their tension. Begin with the face, and then move to the shoulders, arms, hands, and chest.

When you reach your chest, remember to focus on your heart and lungs. Notice how much slower your breathing becomes. Now, move to your stomach and other organs in your stomach. Finally, work down to your hips, legs and feet. Christensen now suggests going back to your face to make sure that it is still calm and relaxed.

Once you have completed this mental scan of your body, it is time to begin mediation. Sometimes it helps to start your meditation session by chanting a mantra, a phrase that focuses your attention. Christensen suggests the word om, pronounced "ohm." Repeat this silently for about a minute to help draw attention from your body to your mind.

Now lie quietly. Thoughts will enter your mind, note them and don't dwell on them. Try to move your thoughts to the edge of your mind, but don't force them. Just let them drift away.

You are trying to find stillness. Your objective is to get your mind quiet, concentrating, and focused. You may not reach this point the first time you attempt to meditate.

Further, when you do reach this point, you may not stay there long. Do not let this upset you. Christensen says, "If you can get one to two minutes of absolute silence, give yourself an A."

Meditate for ten minutes or more, if time permits. Then bring yourself back slowly, repeating the mantra again for about a minute. Don't set an alarm, because this will jar you when it sounds.

The response to meditation in each individual is vastly different. As an example, some feel lighter when they meditate whereas some feel heavier. In the same sense some feel a heightened sense of alertness while others report drowsiness.

However, the body responds, it is a personal, and it is the body's way of learning how to relax.

Unlike the response to meditation, the physical response to poses should be identical amongst most people. Poses have been developed to stretch and strengthen specific muscles while also improving posture and the skeletal system.

Together, the poses are powerful weapons against disease. They make your body more resistant and ready to heal itself.

Of the poses suggested above, the corpse pose is the best pose to end a session on. Nancy Ford-Hohne, founder-director of the Yoga and Health Studies Center in Alexandria, Virginia, suggests thinking to yourself, "Inhale energy and healing, exhale fatigue and stress."

SUMMARY

Alternative health care is an industry that is consistently moving from strength to strength across America. The reasons for that statement holding true appear to be in the growing frustration of the costs and the difficulty accessing quality medical care in the traditional sphere. To mitigate the ill will toward allopathic treatments, a large number of individuals are now seeking alternative remedies to common conditions.

We can all take a leaf out of the book of those that are embracing the different holistic options available, because the lifestyle provides general health and wellbeing benefits and supplements the measures people take to increase their longevity (like diets, exercise and supplements).

The common theme of holistic healing is one of de-stress. As is the case with sexual dysfunction and a range of other conditions stress can cause, prevents improvements or worsens conditions without the proper treatment. In the holistic world, vitamins, herbs and meditation and yoga techniques work to improving the balance of the mind and limiting the build up of stress.

Alternative practitioners confess that this approach is not for everyone. According to Dr. David Edelberg, M.D., a medical director of the American Holistic Center/Chicago, "There are plenty of people who think 'I don't want to change my life. I don't want to hear that my job is giving me a coronary. Just give me a pill for it.'" For these individuals, it is best to go back to your conventional physicians, who will probably do just that.

But the key thing to take out of this report, is that alternative medicine has a place in treating erectile dysfunction and other conditions. In today's society the proactive approach to medicine and fighting ailments is often the most successful as it displays willingness and a desire to 'win' the health battle.

The report has explained in detail the causes of erectile dysfunction and some of the more traditional treatments available. Then, in length we've gone into the alternative treatments, which can be equally as successful. These included stress-relieving techniques such as yoga, meditation and relaxation, as well as approaches with herbs, foods, vitamins and oils.

Despite the difficult psychological effects of erectile dysfunction, it's another psychological response that can lead you on your way to recovery. Quite simply that response, is to take control of your medicine and consider alternatives, which may be as simple as changing your diet and embracing new herbs.

Resources

Learn More

Visit MensGrowth.com to check out the latest advice for men who are looking to be ambitious... Master their lifestyle... Perform in the bedroom... Experience better health, wealth and personal growth...
www.MensGrowth.com

Newsletter

Sign up to MensGrowth.com newsletter to get strategies for better health, increased wealth, style, sex and personal growth news to your inbox. **www.MensGrowth.com/join**

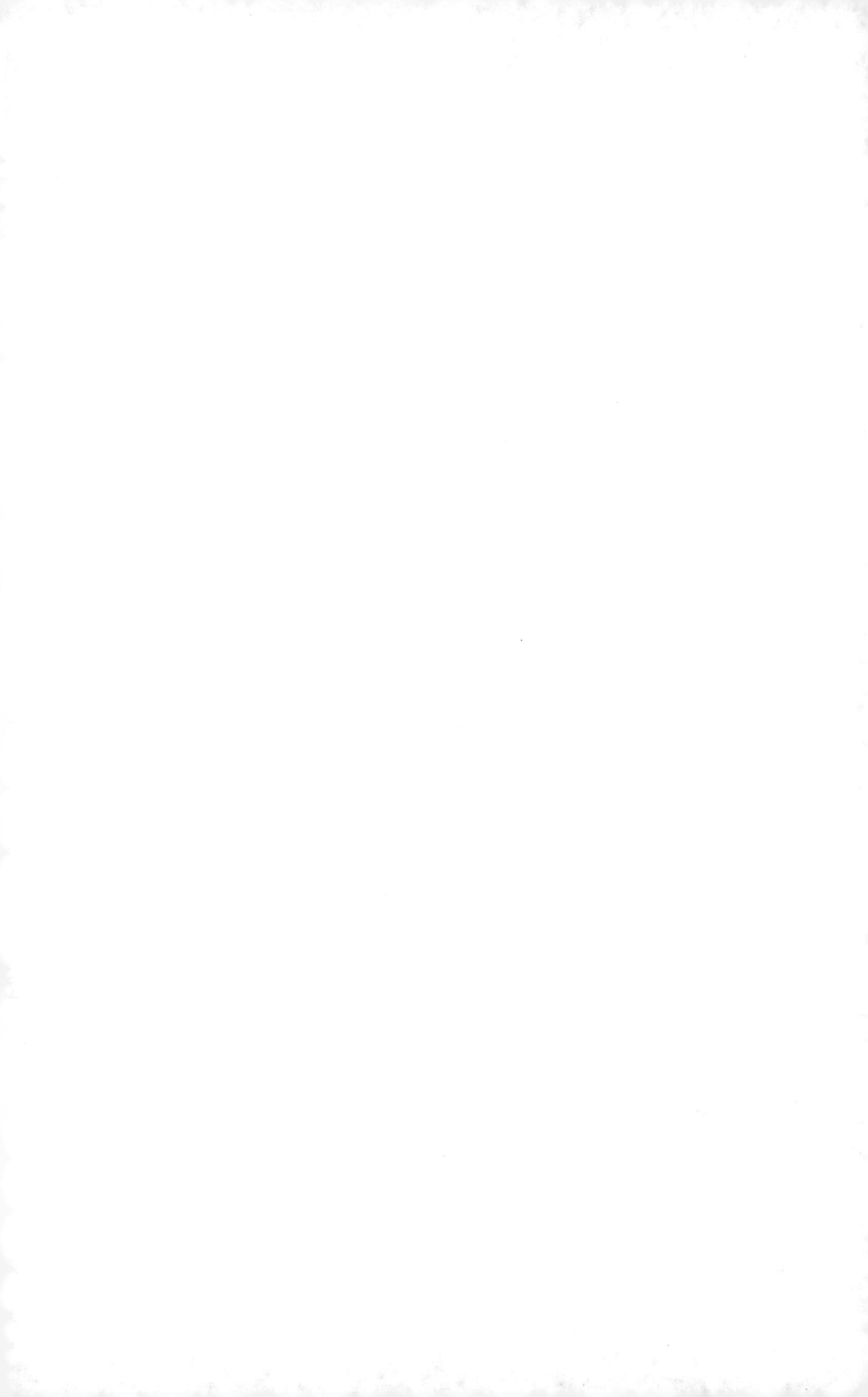